GREEN SMOOTHIES WEIGHT LOSS RECIPES

SARA & MARIA BERN

Published by: Golden Opportunity
Printed by: CreateSpace.com
Editor: Elisabeth Hall

ISBN: 978-91-981872-0-5

Attention You with Eagle Eyes: We've had a number of people proof read this book before we released it to you, however there is a chance you might spot something that was missed. If you find a typo or other obvious error, please send it to us. And if you're the first one to report it we'll send you a free gift! Email your correction to: Sara@A-Golden-Opportunity.com and mark the mail: "Corrections on Green Smoothies – Weight Loss Recipes".

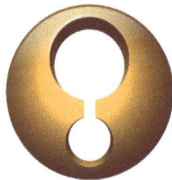

www.A-Golden-Opportunity.com

Golden Opportunity's specialties are
Personal Leadership, Change Management and Wellness

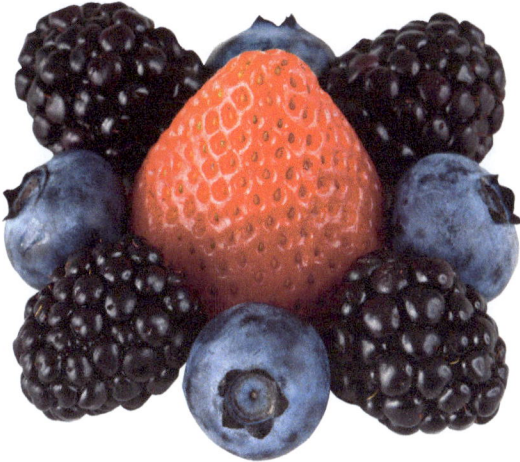

This book is dedicated to **Siv Nordin**, Sara's stepmother, who has inspired and taught us so much about food and nutrients over the years.

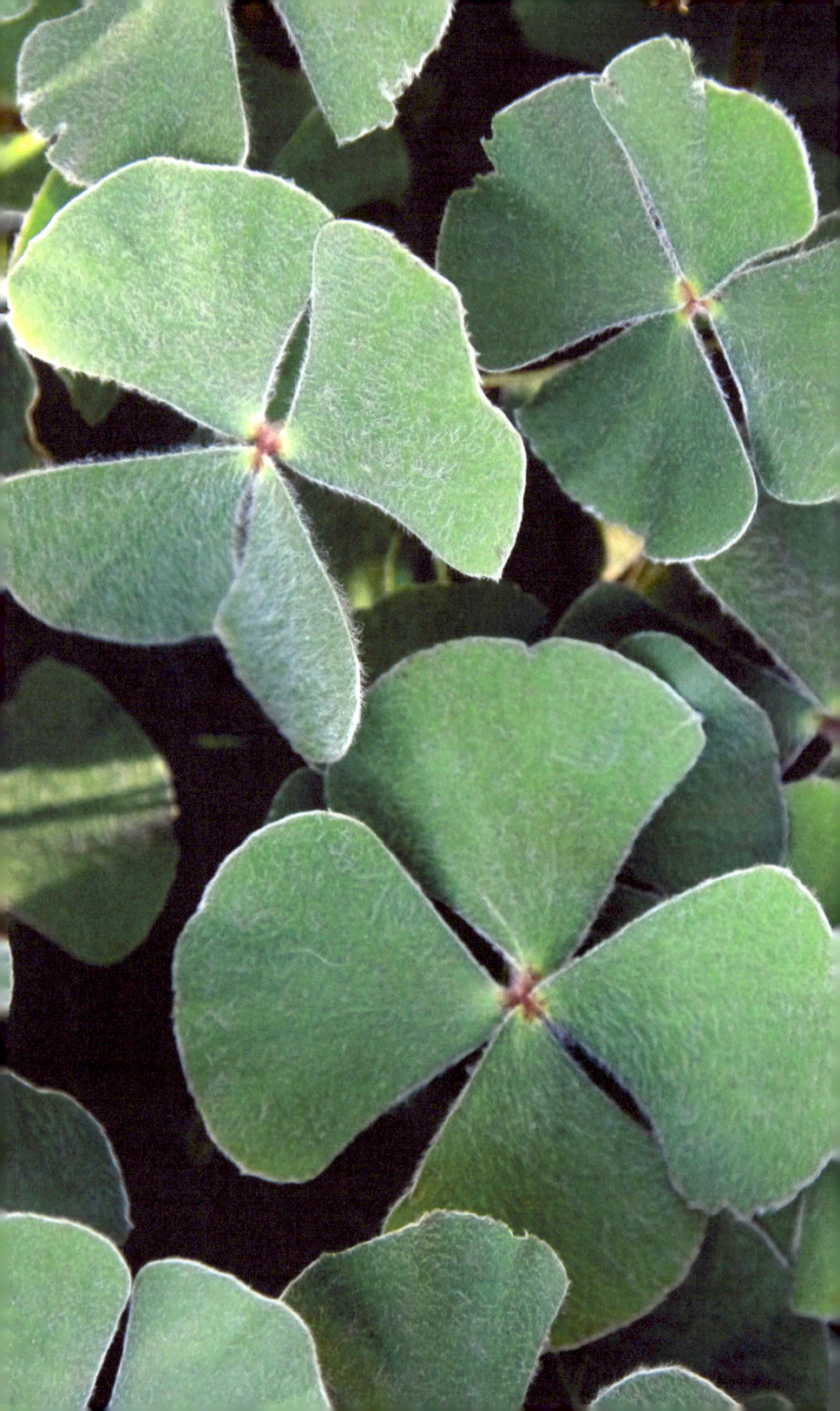

CONTENTS

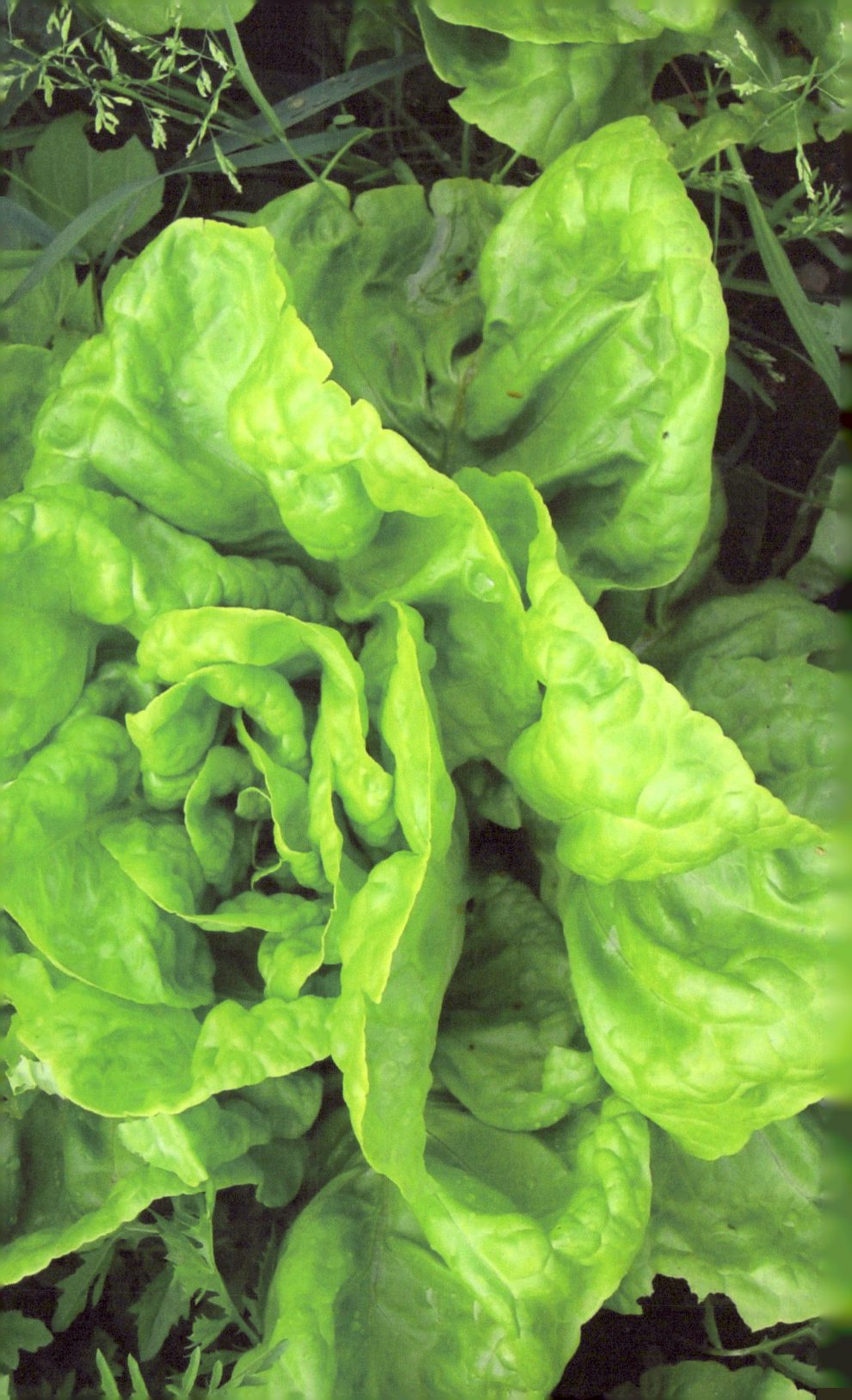

ACKNOWLEDGMENTS

We want to thank **Victoria Boutenko** and
her daughter coming to Sweden to present this topic.
Without that and their contribution to research,
this book with recipes of green smoothies
would never have been created.

Thank you **Caroline Nielsen,** for bringing me to
the Green Smoothie presentation by Victoria.

Thank you **Kim and David McKay,
Elisabeth and Howard Hall and Bernadette
Casinabe** for reviewing our material.

Thanks especially to **Mats Bern**, husband and father,
for his unwavering support and belief in this project.

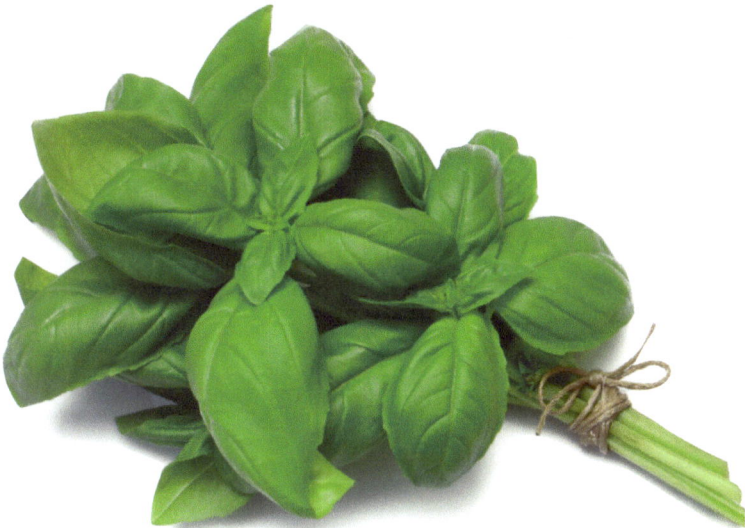

OUR OWN EXPERIENCE

My family started drinking healthy green smoothies in the summer of 2011. One of the reasons I began drinking green smoothies was to lose weight.

During my 3 pregnancies, I had gained 44 pounds and had lost only 16 of them afterwards.

A year after starting drinking green smoothies I was 28 pounds lighter, back to pre-pregnancy weight again and I have been able to keep that weight off, with ease!

28 pounds

108 pounds

Aside from the green smoothies, the rest of my diet is just as before. I can eat anything I like as long as I drink my green smoothies.

In addition to my substantial weight loss, it is now easy for me to keep colds at bay. My body is in a generally good shape.

My daughter, Maria, kept getting colds and had a runny nose basically all the time. After green smoothies on a regular basis, she gets hardly any colds at all, and if she does, she recovers fast.

My husband, Mats, loves having tasty green smoothies from the fridge when returning from his regular tennis practices. It has made diet options easy. Green smoothies provide natural refreshment and serves as an excellent recovery drink.

My daughter Maria and I wrote this book because we want to share with you some of the many delicious recipes for green smoothies we have made and enjoyed over the years.

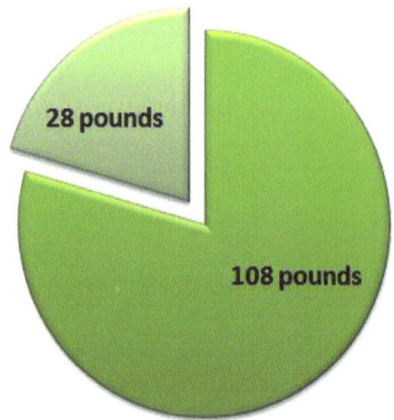

For each smoothie, we would write the ingredients on a little yellow sticky note, helping us remember them when the rest of the family wanted to know what was in the smoothie this time.

On the same yellow sticky notes, we also collected comments and opinions from family and friends who enjoyed these smoothies. These yellow sticky notes are the foundation of this book. Maria helped me to digitalize the notes and to find images. It has been a pure joy for me to add the rest.

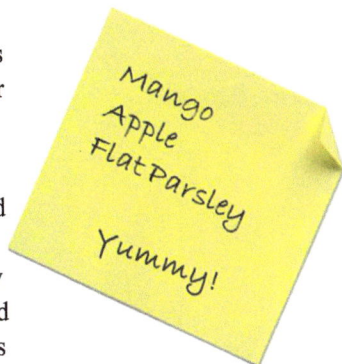

Mango
Apple
Flat Parsley

Yummy!

WE ALSO MADE PEACE WITH WEEDS...

An unexpected bonus effect with green smoothies is that we have finally made peace with the weed that threatens to take over our garden.

For years, I fought in vain against the aggressive ground elder weed.

I know now that the ground elder weed (that I used to hate) is absolutely delicious in the smoothies, as well as in regular salads! We love it!

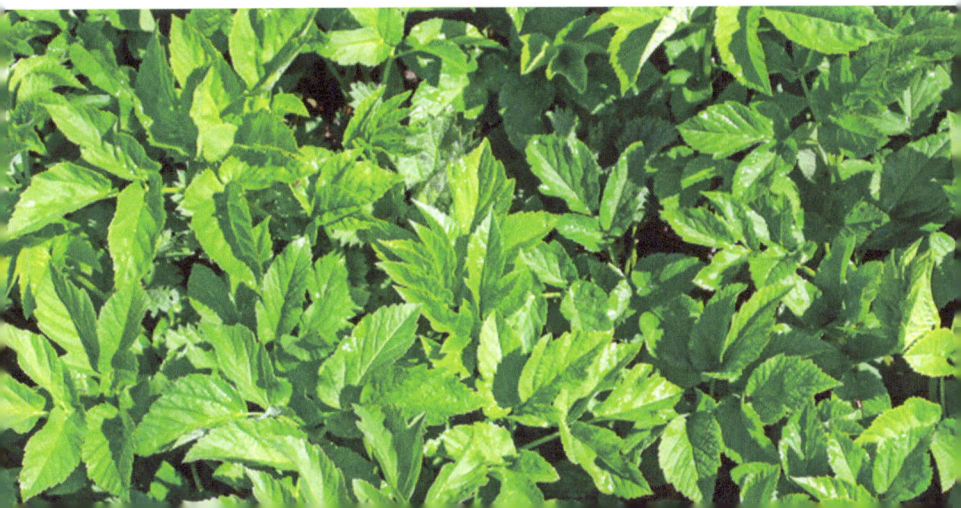

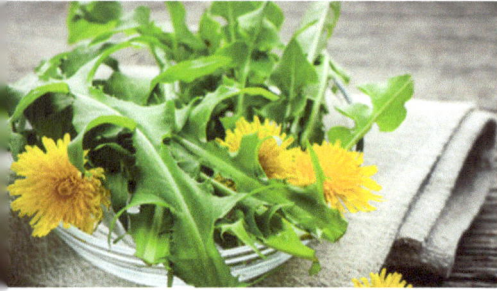

Dandelions are children's delight and many parent's headache in the garden!

How many of you have fought the good fight against dandelions?

Try the young dandelion leaves, they taste very similar to arugula.

Another weed I have fought fiercely over the years is lamb's quarter (Chenopodium album[1]), as they threatened to take over my wild raspberry garden.

Lamb's quarter also tastes a bit like arugula.

You may also try plantain in your green smoothie.

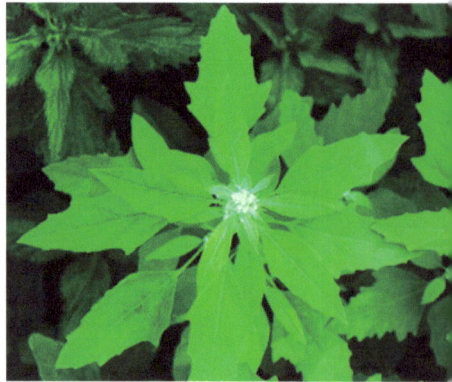

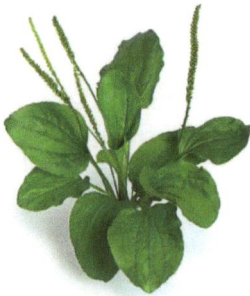

Now, instead of kneeling on all fours weeding our garden, we have time to go for a walk, or go to the gym and get a proper workout.

We certainly hope that you will enjoy green smoothies as much as we do!

Sara and Maria Bern

---

1 Chenopodium album has many names. It is also known as: lamb's quarter, melde, white goosefoot, nickel greens, dungweed, bathua, chandali, chandaliya, fat hen, or pigweed.

HOW IT ALL STARTED

In the summer of 2011, I went to hear a lecture by Victoria Boutenko, author of *Green for Life*, and her daughter. She spoke of how in 1994, she and her entire family suffered from serious health problems (juvenile diabetes, obesity, hyper thyroid, chronic fatigue, arrhythmia, arthritis, asthma as well as allergies). The family switched to a green healthy way of eating, and the entire family was able to completely reverse their health symptoms. They all returned to vibrant health. **WOW!** I was completely flabbergasted.

Victoria had studied wild chimpanzees, whose DNA is nearly identical to human, and had also begun to examine the nutritional content and health benefits of a diet rich in green leafy plant nutrients.

The diet of wild chimpanzees is around 40% greens and they have an exceptional resistance to cancer, AIDS, hepatitis C and other serious diseases.

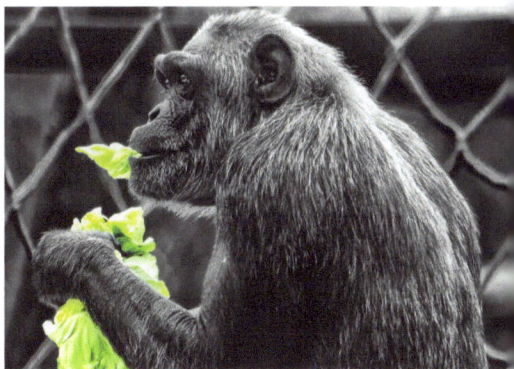

Could the lack of greens be the major cause of modern man's illness, she wondered? And if we can improve our health by eating leaves and greens, what is an easy and appetizing way to do it? By blending greens with fruit and water Victoria went on to discover just such a way, making it delicious and easier to consume large amounts of greens.

At Victoria's presentation, she presented a great amount of research at her talk, supporting the benefits of green smoothies. There were also people there who attended her last workshop, and they personally testified to their own results. This added even more to the credibility of the concept.

I left the presentation totally fascinated and convinced of the importance and value of this new information, and I was determined to make green smoothies part of my own regular diet. When I learned that green smoothies plus some additional omega-3 in the rest of my diet would give me all the nutrition I would need, even proteins, I was even more convinced.

ALL NUTRIENTS? YES, EVEN PROTEINS!

Proteins are made up of amino acids. Greens contains amino acids, which makes it easy for your body to produce healthy proteins suited for the human body.

Green smoothies are able to release the amino acids from the greens because of the blending, a process similar to how cows get proteins from their diet by continually chewing their greens.

How common is it for parents to nag their children:

Chew your food properly! At least 20 times each mouthful!

Who has time for that? Not me! I'm not a cow!

Good news: This time-consuming chewing can be achieved by other means. It's called a blender! It takes less than 5 minutes to make a pitcher of green smoothie.

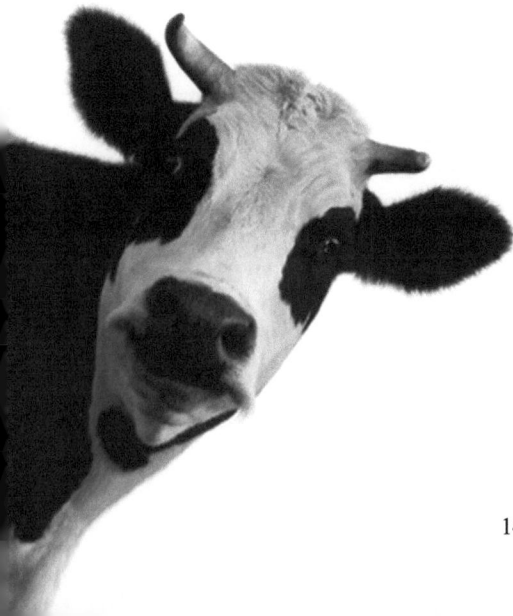

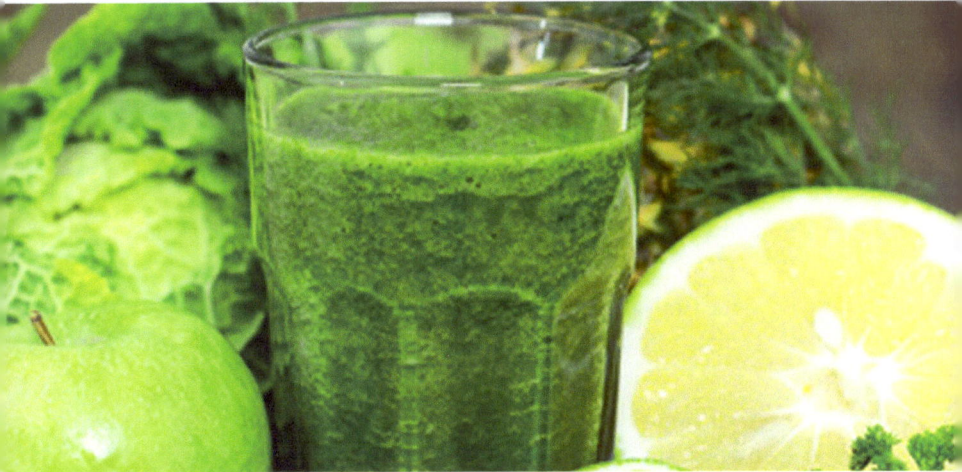

With a blender you get a lot more food down to 1-2 mm sizes, which is what the body needs for proper digestion of proteins.[i] "Incompletely digested protein fragments may be absorbed into the bloodstream. The absorption of these large molecules contributes to the development of food allergies and immunological disorders", Professor W. A. Walker from the Department of Nutrition at the Harvard School of Public Health said.[ii]

Tests have proven that oxidation is slower in blended smoothies, compared to juices. A green smoothie can stay fresh in the refrigerator for 2 or 3 days.

I learned of Victoria that a vegetarian diet high in raw vegetables was also optimal for cancer patients as long as it was supplemented with omega-3 fats and contained enough calories to be healthy. Green smoothies contains chlorophyll, which is very similar to human blood molecules.

Dr. Ann Wigmore use to say: *"Consuming chlorophyll is like receiving a healthy blood transfusion"*.

Green smoothies are a complete food, compared to juices, because they contain fiber.

HOW DO THEY REDUCE WEIGHT?

Green smoothies help weight loss primarily by improving metabolism and decreasing sweet cravings.

* **Improving metabolism** means that the body's cells can take up nutrients and expel waste products more easily and efficiently.

* **Green smoothies are a lighter snack** than e.g. sandwiches and cookies, that are likely to increase your weight.

* **Your sugar cravings and cravings for sweets will diminish** step by step when you include green smoothies in your diet and you will start to appreciate more flavors. Since sugar usually ends up as body fat, reducing sugar is a major component in weight loss.

In the Green Smoothies Recipes chapter we have also added notes showing how individual fruits help your weight reduction.

How much weight you will lose will vary depending on where you start and how much of your current diet you exchange for green smoothies. One or two liters per day of green smoothies is a sustainable, safe and fun way of losing excess weight.

You may think the way I did; *"Yeah, yeah, here is another diet that will make me lose weight but will not provide me with all the nutrition I need. This may not be a sustainable diet"*. Well, I was wrong!

THEY CONTAIN BASICALLY ALL NUTRIENTS

Victoria Boutenko collaborates with nutrition experts at the prestigious Karolinska Institute in Stockholm, Sweden, where the scientists confirm this.

Omega-3 fats taken in combination with green smoothies makes the diet complete from a nutritional perspective. To get the omega-3 oils that you need you can add flax seeds, chia, or other omega-3 rich foods.

Research shows that if you have the right balance of omega-3, versus omega-6 oils it is much easier to maintain your proper weight.[iii]

NOTE: Do not add seeds, nuts and other ingredients directly into your green smoothie though, as they may slow down the uptake of nutrients.

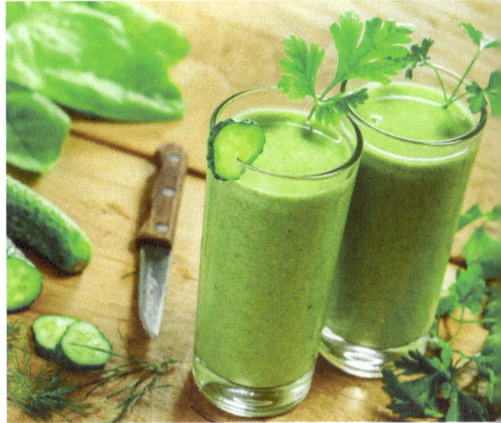

One liter of green smoothies per day is enough to maintain good health.

Should you want to work on reversing diseases of different kinds, Victoria Boutenko recommends increasing your intake of green smoothies to 2 liters a day.

HOW TO MAKE GREEN SMOOTHIES

Most systems work best if they are kept simple rather than made complex; simplicity should thus be the key goal. We have chosen to use that very principle in our recipes too.

PROCEDURE

- **Put fruits and / or berries into a mixer**
- **Add greens**
- **Add 1-2 cups of water (or coconut milk)**
- **Mix it smooth.**

THAT'S IT!
Serve and enjoy with a beautiful decoration!

Make enough of what you can consume for the day in the morning and keep it cold. We suggest that you drink your smoothie slowly and allow it to mix with your saliva.

WHAT GREENS TO USE

There are a wide variety of things which work as greens for these recipes.

Chlorophyll does not only give the green its color but also provides numerous health benefits! The important thing is that they contain proteins and chlorophyll[iv].

Some examples of greens would be:

- lettuce of all kinds, grass, ground elder, lamb's quarter, beet leaves, parsley, purslane, spinach, Swiss chard, amaranth leaves and sorrel. Sweet baby-leaf spinach is fine to eat in quantity. Even tree leaves, like birch leaves, are edible.

GREENS: With very few exceptions, greens are the flat leaves of a plant, attached to the stem, which can be wrapped around one finger.

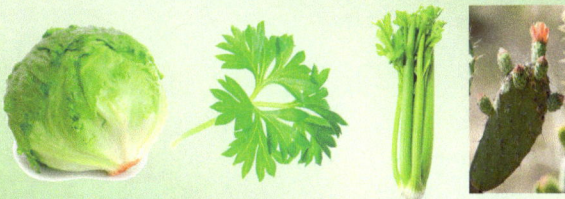

NOTE: Celery and Nopales cactus leaves and also counts as greens.

Make sure that you rotate the greens you are using. Almost all greens contain very small amounts of alkaloids. Some alkaloids will strengthen the immune system. However, if you keep consuming any type of green for too many weeks without change, eventually the same type of alkaloids may accumulate in your body and cause unwanted poisoning symptoms.

Some greens which are low in oxalic acid and good to eat regularly in green smoothies are dandelion greens and kale (which has more calcium than dairy, by the way), lettuce, celery, turnip greens, carrot tops (yes, you read it correctly), watercress, escarole, mustard greens, broccoli and asparagus. Most other greens fit into this category as well.

A few greens are high in oxalic acid which binds to calcium to form calcium oxalate, an insoluble salt, which can cause kidney stones if taken to excess. Add these to a Green Smoothie once in a while for variety. These high-oxalate greens are lamb's quarter, beet leaves, parsley, purslane, spinach, clover grass, aloe leaf, Swiss chard, amaranth leaves and sorrel. Do not use rhubarb leaves, as they are poisonous when eaten in large quantities.

WHAT FRUITS TO USE

Locally and/or organically grown greens and fruits will give you the best nutrition value. Tree-ripened fruit is best.

Want a creamy smoothie? Banana, mango, avocado and ripe pears all lend a creamier texture to the drink. **Want it less sweet?** As an alternative to the sweet fruits in your green smoothies, feel free to use vegetables with low starch content[2].

These include:
- cucumbers, zucchini, squash, tomatoes, avocado, celery, and peppers.

In reality, both avocado and tomatoes are fruits. They are both known to be good for weight loss.[v]

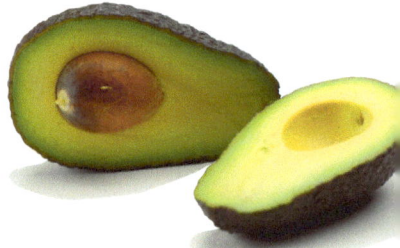

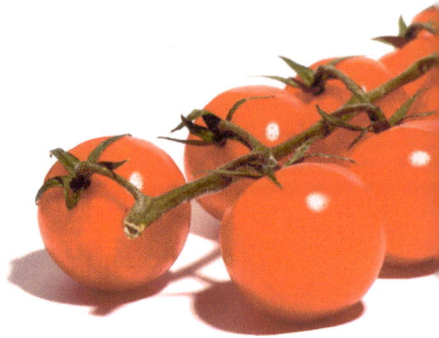

2. The combination of starchy vegetables with fruit may cause fermentation and gas in the stomach. Starchy vegetables to avoid in green smoothies include carrots, beets, broccoli stems, cauliflower, cabbage, brussels sprouts, egg plant, pumpkin, squash, okra, peas, corn, and green beans.

HOW MUCH TO USE?

To be honest the exact amounts of each fruit and each green is not as important as:

- the greens/fruit proportions and
- variety of ingredients.

Try it out and see what fits your taste buds! In the beginning you may start by adding extra fruit to make the smoothies a little sweeter or you may choose to add a bit of honey.

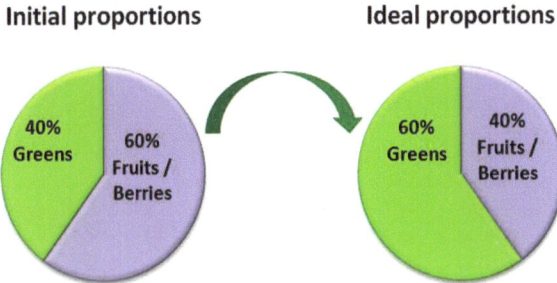

Initial proportions   **Ideal proportions**

40% Greens   60% Fruits / Berries   60% Greens   40% Fruits / Berries

Make your smoothies truly delicious! That way you will always look forward to your next one. If your drink is not tasty for you, you will eventually cease drinking them. So please your taste buds!

As your sweet tooth diminishes, you can increase the percentage of greens and decrease the percentage of fruit. This will become easier over time, as your craving for sugar diminishes and your weight loss journey takes on a new dimension!

TOOLS FOR MAKING THEM

Use any blender to start making green smoothies. A high speed blender will allow continuous use and speed of creation, but any blender will do. There are many inexpensive brands out there. This is the one I use.

If you get hooked on smoothies, we can recommend an investment in a Vita-mix blender. This minimizes preparation time since the Vita-mix easily handles larger chunks. Take an apple for example. You need only to take away the stem and you can add the rest of the apple as is.

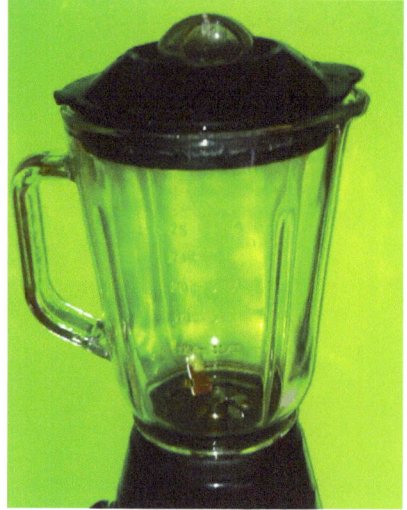

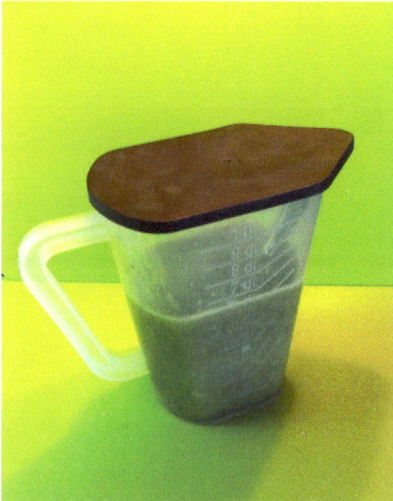

After an initial serving, we like to pour our smoothies into a pitcher with a lid and keep it in the refrigerator for the rest of the day.

The smoothie quickly separates into liquid and pulp, so you may want to leave a spoon in the pitcher for stirring each time you pour yourself a glass.

Green smoothies tend to stick to the glass. Quickly rinse the glasses and the blender after use. Do not leave them dirty in the dishwasher.

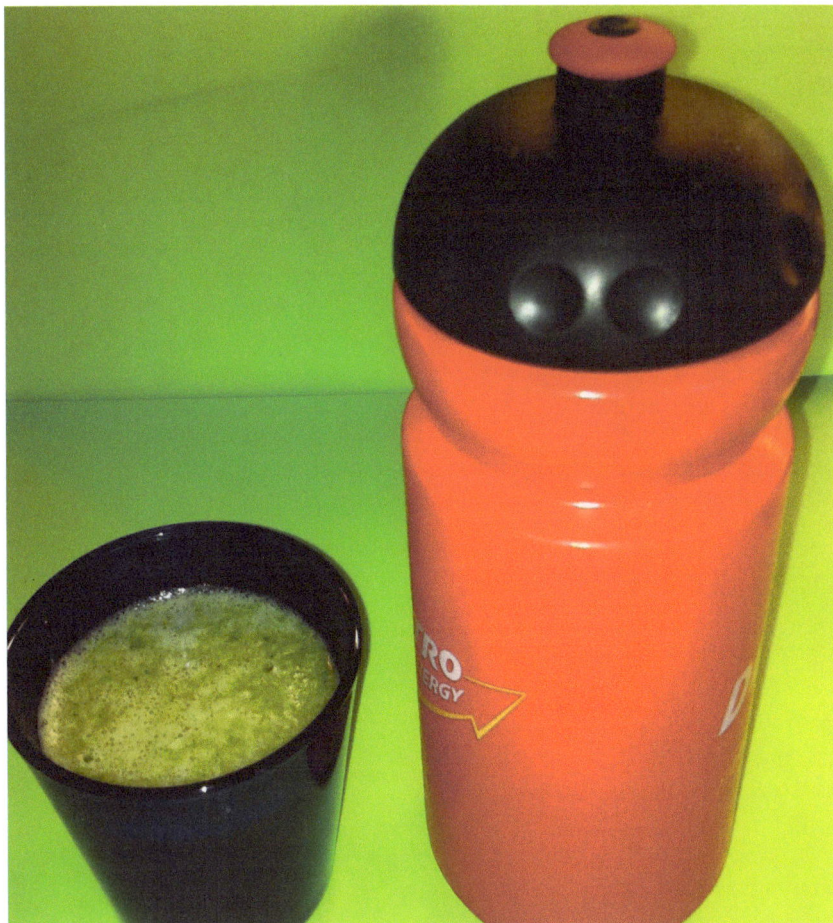

Many people are not used to the color of the green smoothie, and some actually think it looks dreadful. Therefore, we usually use colored glasses for our smoothies, or opaque travel bottles.

I often bring my smoothie to my office in travel bottle or a coffee mug with a lid. This allows me not only to minimize the chance of spilling it, but also to keep it private and not distract others with it.

GREEN SMOOTHIE RECIPES

The recipes intentionally say very little about precise amounts of ingredients since we encourage you to experiment and find your own balance of taste and texture. Remember the 60/40 ratio of greens to fruits as the goal, even if you start out somewhere else.

Add one or two cups of water (e.g. 3-5 deciliter), depending on how thick you want your smoothie to be. This will help the blender work more smoothly. If you forget the liquid, your blender may not want to cooperate at all. We usually blend our smoothies with half of the water. The rest of the water is added when rinsing out the blender.

Note that apples need thorough blending as their peel is very hard.

VARIATION OF THE SMOOTHIES

Our suggested recipes are simple, easy and tasty. You are welcome to play around with them. Before you do, you should read these short notes on how to vary the smoothies, as they will provide some guidance.

Fresh ginger or herbs such as basil, coriander, salvia, thyme, cilantro, and tarragon may add a powerful spicy taste to your smoothie!

Herbs can also be used as a beautiful, inviting garnish!

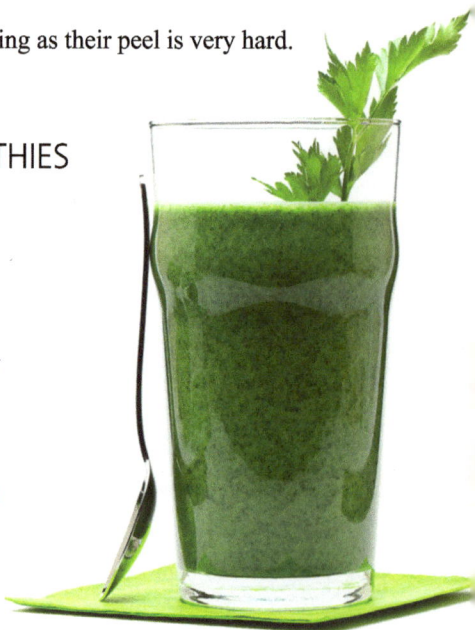

NOTE: If you keep most of your recipes simple you will maximize the nutritional benefits and make it easier to digest your smoothie.

FAT BURNER TIP:
You may exchange all or some of the water in the smoothies for coconut milk. Coconut is botanically a fruit, not a nut.

COCONUT reduces weight because it contains medium chain triglycerides (MCTs) which may increase the liver's rate of metabolism by up to 30 percent.[vi and vii]

Coconut also fills you up so you will probably eat less junk food.

Coconut oil, coconut milk (not the low fat variety), coconut flour, and shredded (unsweetened) coconut all contain MCTs.

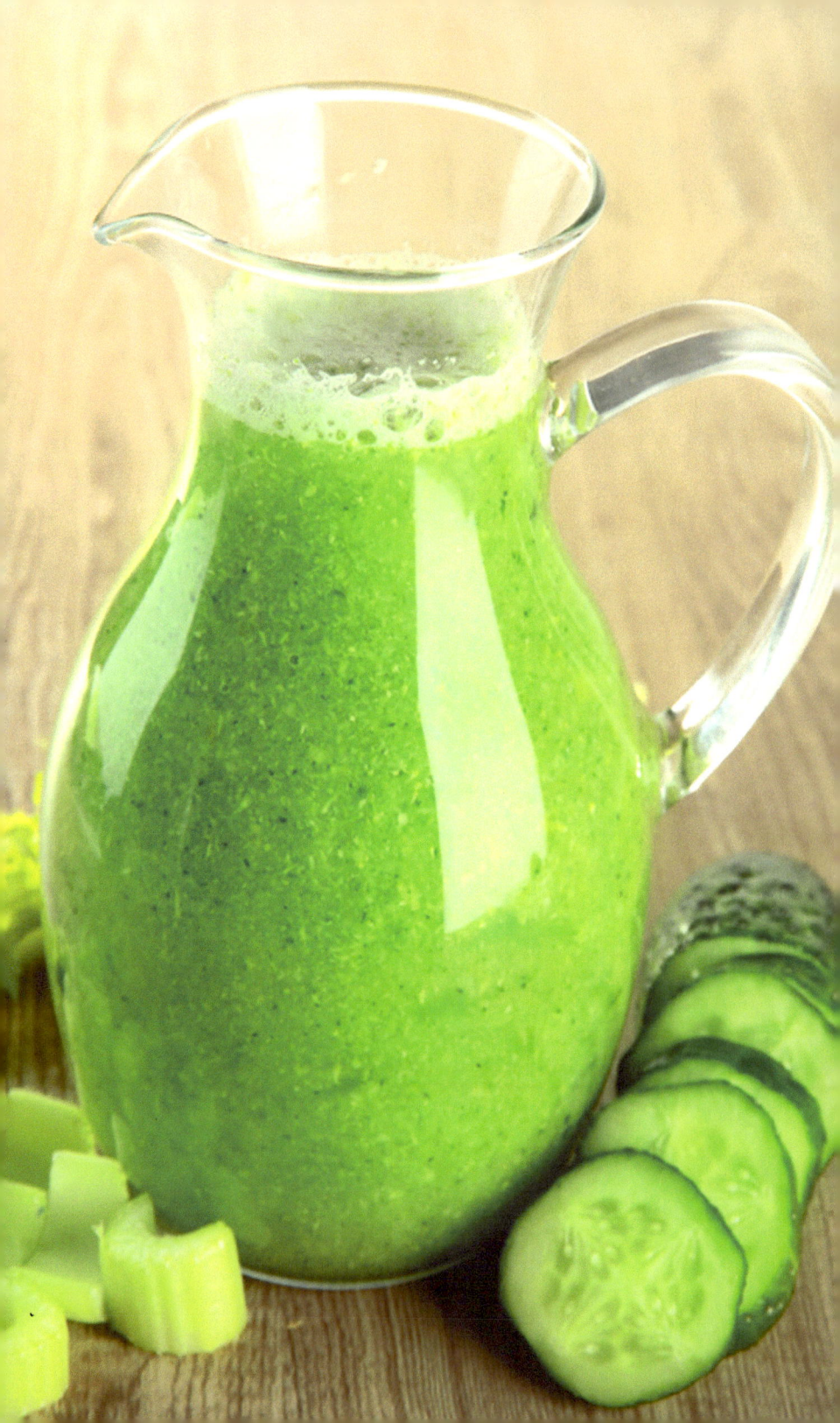

Creamy Smoothie

2 Apples
1 Avocado
Arugula salad
1-2 cups water

Basil Sprinkle

1 Mango
1 Banana
Green leaf lettuce
Corn salad (Mâche)
Some basil leaves
1-2 cups water

Creamy Gazpacho

3 Tomatoes
1 Avocado
Lemon juice to taste
Green leaf lettuce
Chili pepper to taste
A little cilantro
1-2 cups water

Apricot Valley

5 Apricots
1 Orange
½ Lemon
Romaine lettuce
1-2 cups water

AVOCADOS reduce weight since they are full of healthy omega-9 fatty acids which speed the conversion of fat into energy and boost the rate of your metabolism.[viii]

TOMATOES reduce weight since they contain the phytochemical lycopene, which creates the amino acid carnitine,[ix] which burns fat efficiently.

LEMONS reduce weight because they are excellent liver detoxifiers and lemons also alkalize our body.[x]

Lemons may seem acidic based on taste but in the process of being metabolized by the body, they actually alkalize our bodily fluids and tissues. To maintain a healthy liver is also very important for the body's digestion and fat burning ability, since the liver is one of the organs responsible for these functions.

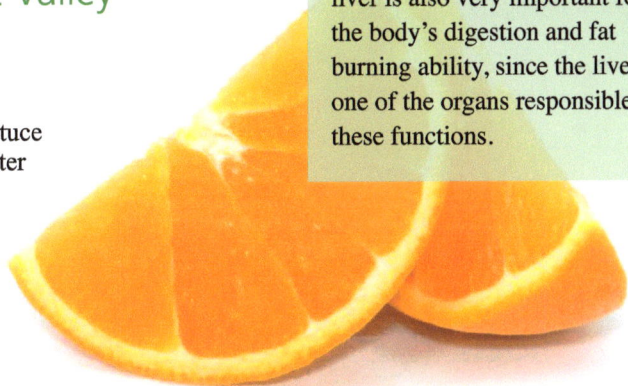

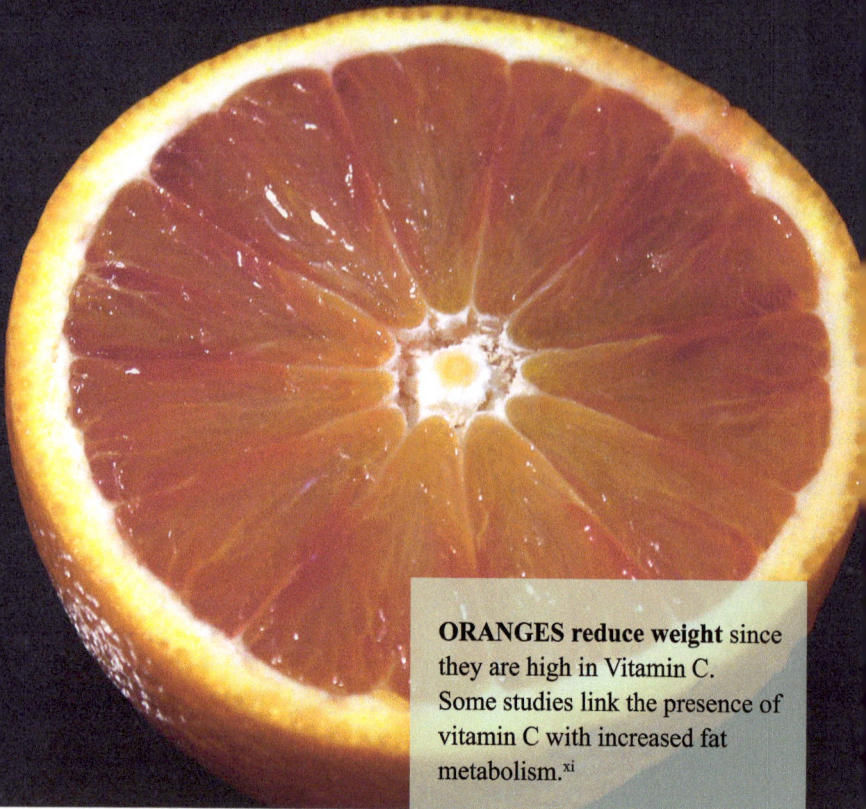

ORANGES reduce weight since they are high in Vitamin C. Some studies link the presence of vitamin C with increased fat metabolism.[xi]

Fantasy Of Taste

1 Banana
2 Blood oranges
Corn salad (Mâche)
1-2 cups water

Sweet Chard

Swiss Chard (Mangold)
1 Banana
1-2 cups water

Fresh Kiwi

1 Blood orange
1 Banana
1 Kiwi
1/3 pot Fresh parsley
1-2 cups water

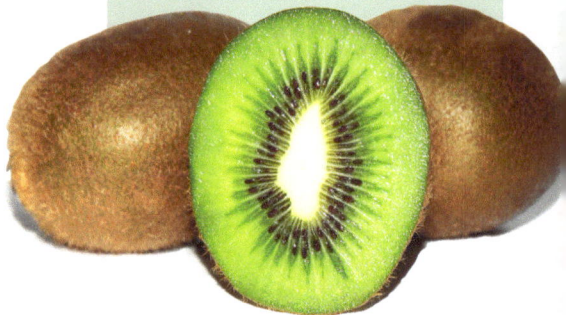

Mango Dream

1 Apple
1/3 Mango
Baby spinach
1-2 cups water

Mango Power

1 Mango
Lamb's quarter
1-2 cups water

Mango Delight

1 Mango
Flat parsley
1-2 cups water

MANGOS reduce weight since they are packed with nutrients and fibers, but very low in calories.

Mangos are rich in minerals and vitamins, but they are sodium free, cholesterol free and essentially fat free.

Studies show that mango seed extracts are excellent weight reducers.[xii]

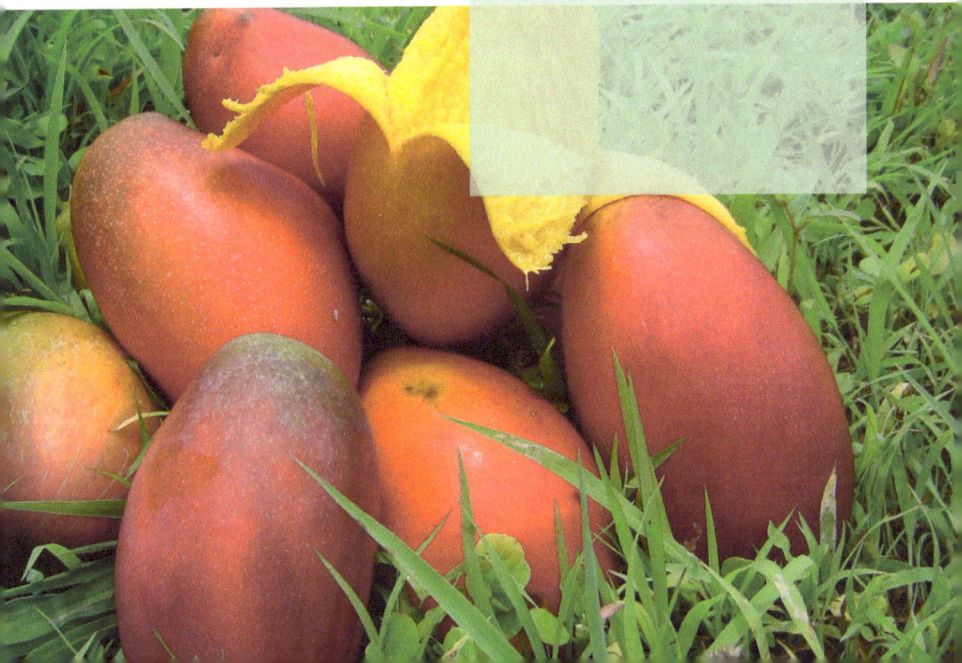

Raspberry Patch

1 Apple
1 Banana
Raspberries
Romaine lettuce
1-2 cups water

Green Berry Blast

1 Banana
Raspberries
Iceberg lettuce
Baby spinach
1-2 cups water

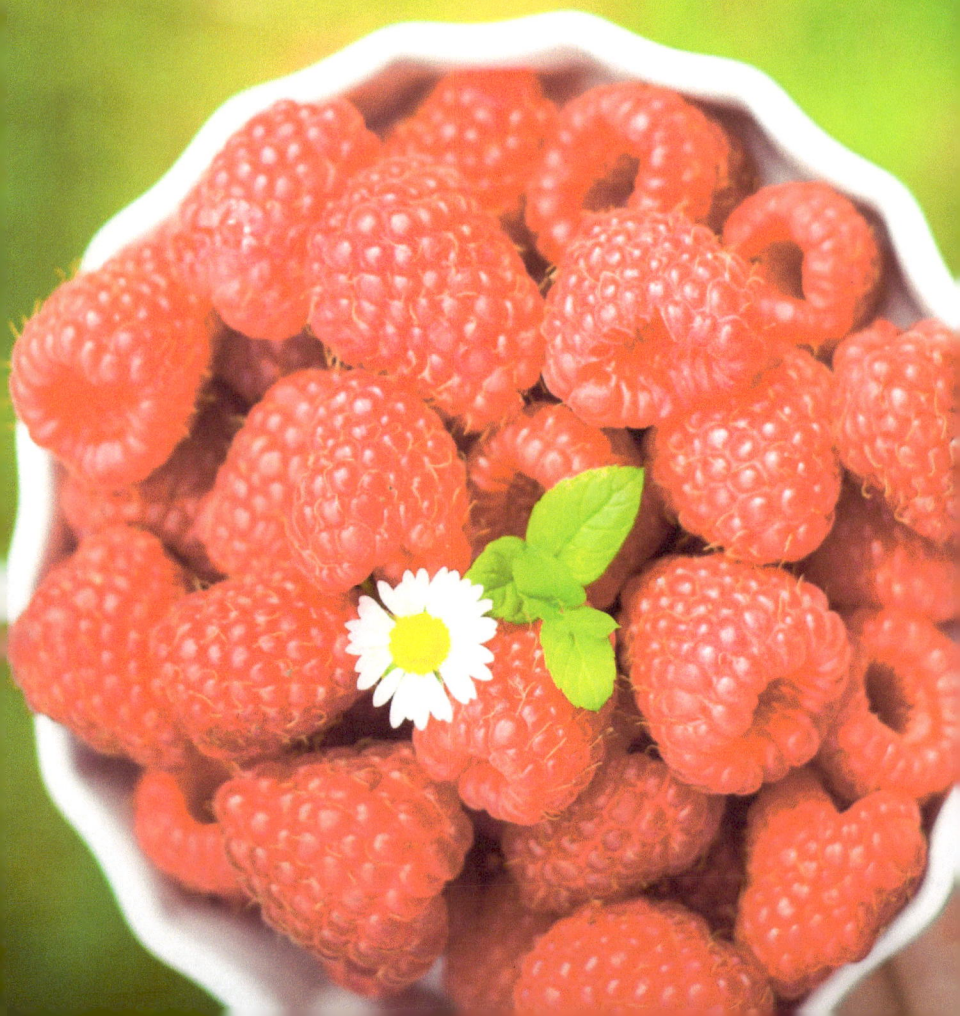

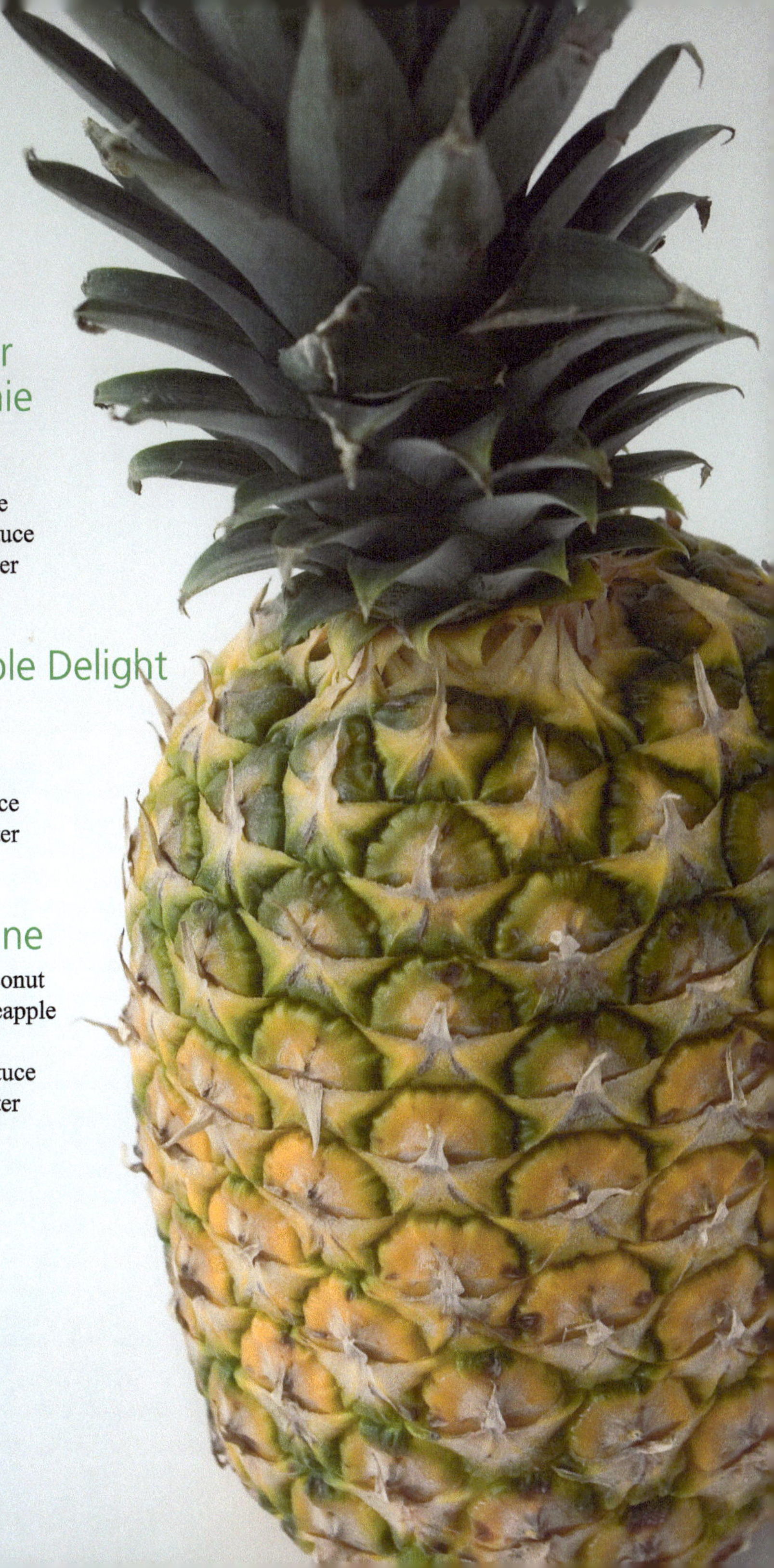

Summer Smoothie

1 Apple
1 Banana
1/5 Pineapple
Romaine lettuce
1-2 cups water

Pineapple Delight

1 Orange
1 Banana
½ Pineapple
Iceberg lettuce
1-2 cups water

Coco Pine

1 young Coconut
½ small Pineapple
1 Pear
Romaine lettuce
1-2 cups water

Think Orange

1 cup Watermelon
1 Orange
1 Apple
½ Banana
Baby spinach
1-2 cups water

Soothing Smoothie

1 cup Watermelon
Green leaf lettuce
1-2 cups water

Nordic Sorrel

1 cup Watermelon
1 Apple
½ Banana
Sorrel (¼ of the greens)
Ground elder (¾ of the greens)
1-2 cups water

Bananas in Pajamas

1 cup Watermelon
1 Orange
½ Banana
1-2 cups water

PINEAPPLES reduce weight since they support your digestion[xiii] and they ease inflammation by removing fat from the stomach and intestines.

Pineapples are also an excellent source of Vitamin C, which in addition to supporting weight loss, also offers protection from the flu.

WATERMELONS reduce weight since they contain the amino acid arginine that may enhance the metabolism according to a new study in the *Journal of Nutrition*.

Adding arginine to the diet enhances the oxidation of fat and glucose and increases lean muscle.

Banana Tree

1 cup Watermelon
1 Banana
½ cup Alfalfa sprouts
1-2 cups water

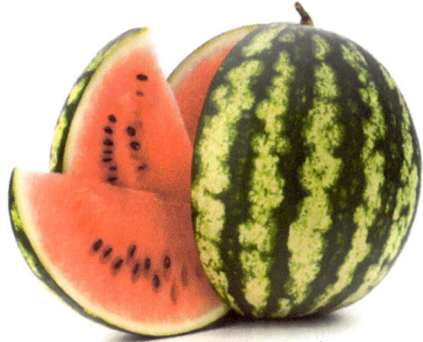

Romantic Sunset

1 Papaya
1 Orange
Romaine lettuce
1-2 cups water

Alfalfa Smoothie

1 Banana
Romaine lettuce
½ cup Alfalfa sprouts
Arugula
1-2 cups water

Alfa Power

1 Banana
1 cup Watermelon
1 Pear (ripe)
½ cup Alfalfa sprouts
Flat Parsley
1-2 cups water

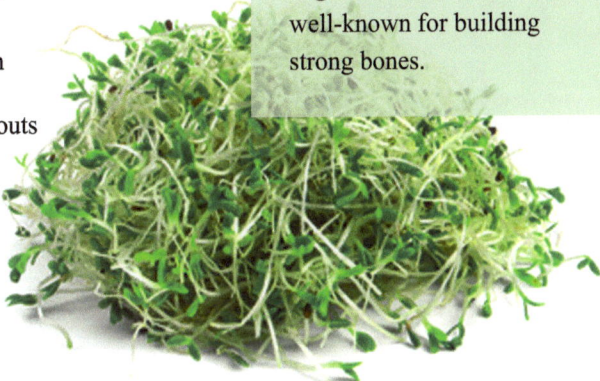

**ALFALFA SPROUTS
reduce weight** due to their
nutrient content.

Alfalfa sprouts have all the
essential amino acids and all
important vitamins.

They are especially good
for our kidneys and bladder,
writes Paul Pitchford in *Healing With Whole Foods*. Also
well-known for building
strong bones.

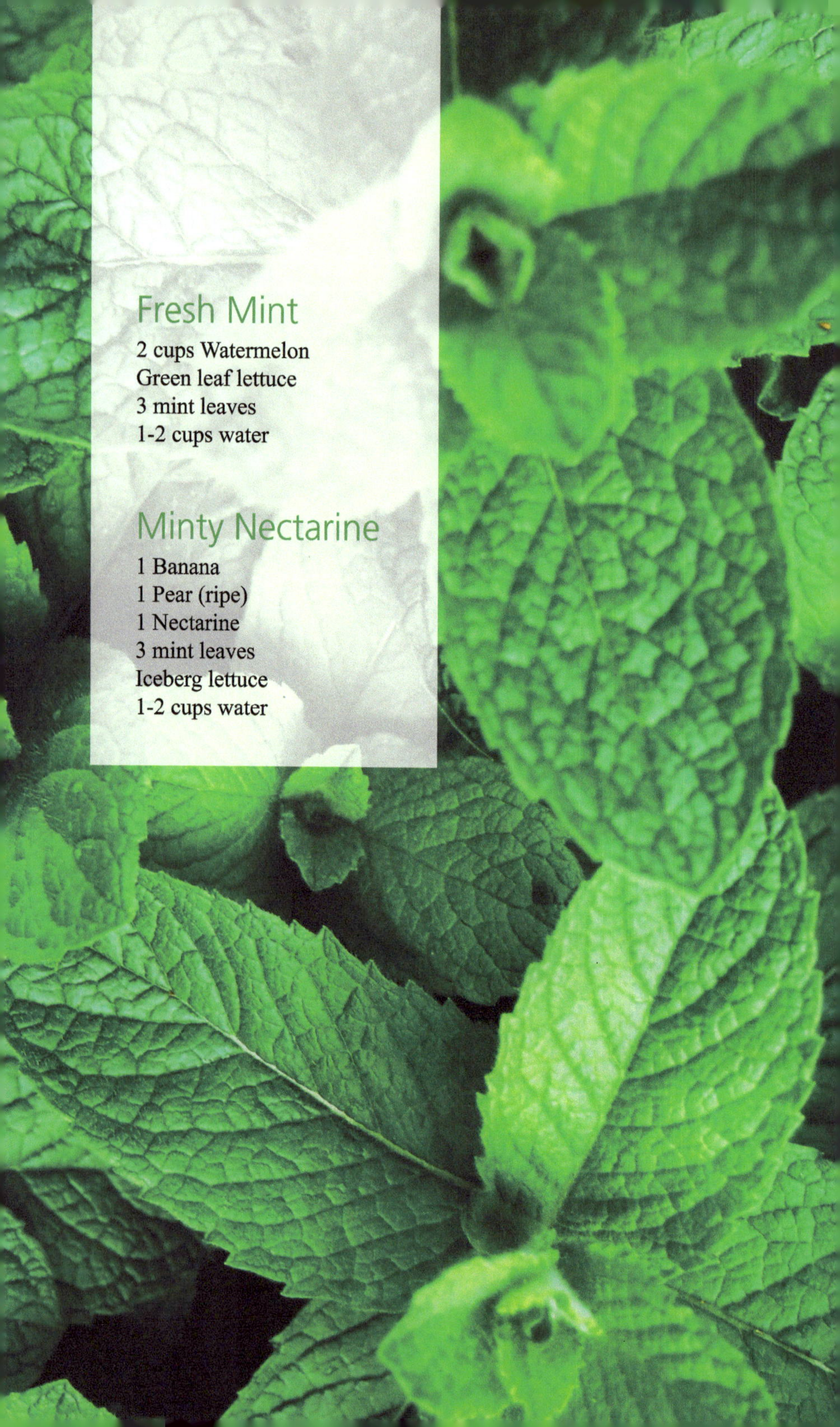

Fresh Mint

2 cups Watermelon
Green leaf lettuce
3 mint leaves
1-2 cups water

Minty Nectarine

1 Banana
1 Pear (ripe)
1 Nectarine
3 mint leaves
Iceberg lettuce
1-2 cups water

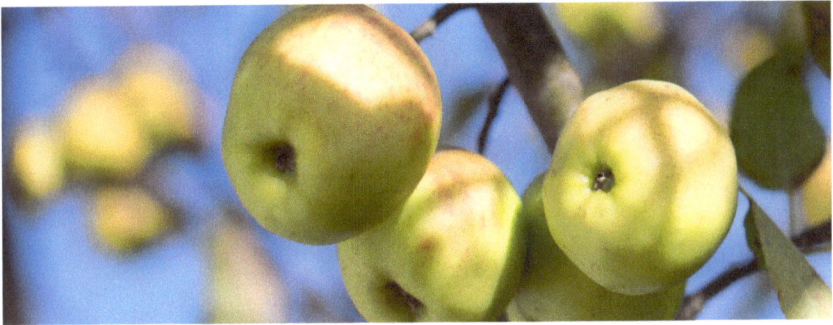

Banana Dance

1 Banana
Green leaf lettuce
1/3 pot Fresh Parsley
1-2 cups water

Garden Smoothie

2 Bananas
Cascade or Summer crisp lettuce
Ground elder
1-2 cups water

Sweat Pears

1 Mango
1 Pear (ripe)
Iceberg lettuce
1-2 cups water

Fruit Cascade

1 Nectarine
1 Banana
Cascade or Summer crisp lettuce
1-2 cups water

Magical Apples

1/2 Mango
1 Apple
A handful Fresh Parsley
1-2 cups water

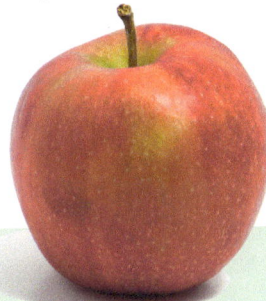

APPLES reduce weight
because they are high in fiber
which helps weight loss in two
ways. First you quickly get full,
which prompts the body to stop
eating.

Second, fiber also prevents
constipation, and by stimulating
the elimination process, it helps
to remove body fat.

Romantic Apple

1 Apple
1 cup Watermelon
1 Banana
1 Orange
Romaine lettuce
1-2 cups water

Dream of Pears

Romaine lettuce
1 Banana
1 Pear (ripe)
1-2 cups water

Currant Deluxe

1/6 Water melon
1 ½ Banana
¼ cup Black currants
A handful Fresh Parsley
1-2 cups water

Fruit Power

1/6 Watermelon
1 Nectarine
Green leaf lettuce
1-2 cups water

Desert Dessert

1 Banana
1 Cactus leave
Green leaf lettuce
Iceberg lettuce
1-2 cups water

Baby Banana

1 Banana
1 Apple
Baby spinach
1-2 cups water

Baby Laughter

1 Banana
Arugula
Baby spinach
Red lettuce
1-2 cups water

BANANAS reduce weight since they are high in resistant starch,[xiv] a type of fiber found in carbohydraterich foods, that enhances fat burning.

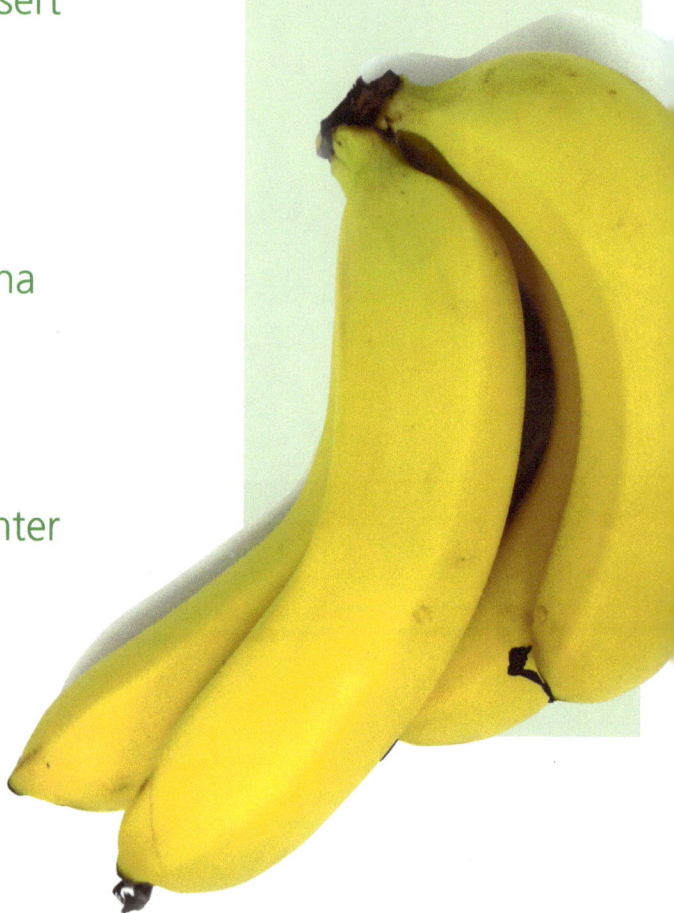

Strawberry Sunset

1 Banana
Strawberries
Fresh Parsley
Romaine lettuce
1-2 cups water

King of the Garden

1 Mango
Ground elder
1-2 cups water

Romantic Currant

1 Mango
1 Banana
¼ cup Black currants
Romaine lettuce
1-2 cups water

Lean Rainbow

1 Grapefruit
1 Banana
Rainbow chard
1-2 cups water

Bittersweet Grape

1 Red grapefruit
Romaine lettuce
1-2 cups water

STRAWBERRIES reduce weight since a cup of strawberries only contains 50 calories and 7 grams of sugar. Still, it provides 3 grams of fiber which helps your digestion.

BERRIES reduce weight due to several factors. They satisfy your sweet/sugar cravings and have a very impressive nutrient profile.

GRAPEFRUITS reduce weight by lowering the blood sugar and the related feelings of hunger. Many studies confirm that grapefruit is an excellent weight loss food.[xv] In one study at Johns Hopkins University, women who eat grapefruit daily shed almost 20 pounds on average in only 13 weeks, without changing anything else in their diet or lifestyle.

Blueberry Hill

¼ cup Blueberries
1 Orange
Spinach leaves
1-2 cups water

Refreshing Blues

½ cup Blueberries
1 Pear
Rainbow Chard
Purple Kale
Grated fresh Ginger to taste
1-2 cups water

BLUEBERRIES reduce weight by reducing abdominal fat,[xvi] the kind of fat linked to increased waist size and increased risk for diabetes and heart disease.

Researchers from the Texas Woman's University (TWU) also found that **BLUEBERRIES have a significant impact on weight reduction** efforts and obesity since they inhibit the creation of new fat cells by altering lipid metabolism.[xvi]

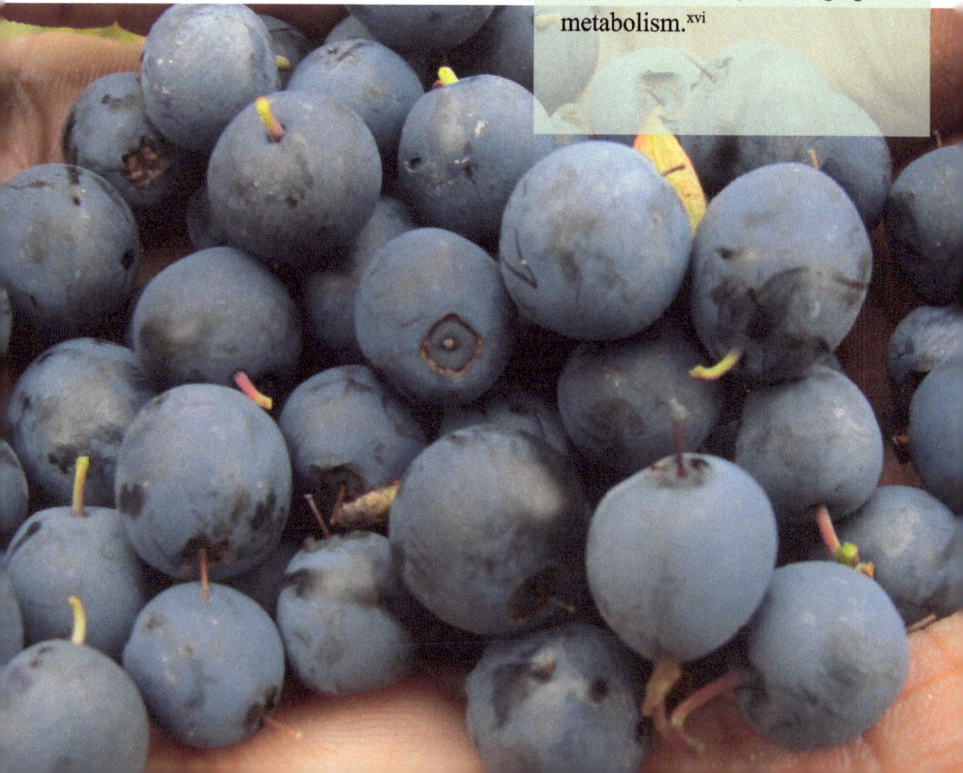

Drop Tropical

3 Persimmon (Also called Sharon or Kaki)
1 Grapefruit
Baby spinach
1-2 cups water

Persimmon Sharon

3 Persimmon (Sharon/Kaki)
Baby spinach
1-2 cups water

Diospyros Kaki Sharon

5 Persimmon (Sharon/Kaki)
¼ Lemon
Baby spinach
1-2 cups water

Tropical Mix

1 Persimmon (Sharon/Kaki)
1 Mandarin orange
1 Mango
Baby spinach
1-2 cups water

Aloe Fresh

1 Aloe leaf
Baby spinach
1 Banana
Lemon juice to taste
1-2 cups water

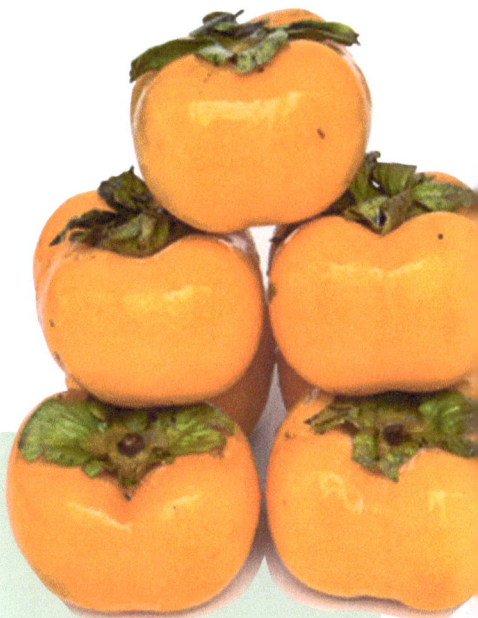

PERSIMMONS (Sharon/ Kaki) reduce weight through, among other things, a very high fiber content. It is high in Vitamin C and A.

The persimmon's very high proportion of betacarotene (pro-vitamin A) makes it nutritionally valuable.

Persimmons are said to be helpful against stomach ailments and diarrhea.

Apple Sunset

1 Apple
1 Banana
Ground elder
1-2 cups water

Think Green

1 Apple
1 Peach or Nectarine
Ground elder
1-2 cups water

Lamb's Quarter Smoothie

1 Banana
1 Apple
Lamb's quarter
1-2 cups water

Fresh Coco

1 Apple
1 Lemon
Corn salad (Mâche)
1 cup Coconut milk

Sweet Coco

1 Mango
1 Pear
A sprinkle of Lemon
Baby Spinach
1 cup Coconut milk

Lemon Grass Walk

1 Banana
1 Apple
Iceberg lettuce
1 Lemon grass straw
1-2 cups water

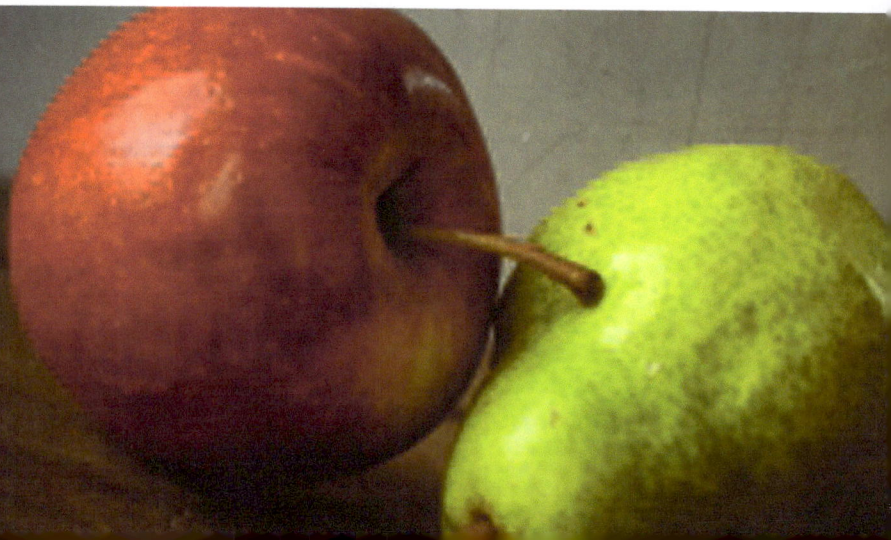

ABOUT THE AUTHORS

SARA BERN

Sara lives with her husband Mats, three children, and two cats in Huddinge, a suburb of Stockholm, the capital of Sweden.

After a long international career in telecommunications and IT, she now works as an executive coach and change management consultant.

Her websites include:
www.A-Golden-Opportunity.com
www.BecomingAGoalAchiever.com
www.EmotionalFreedomTechnique.biz

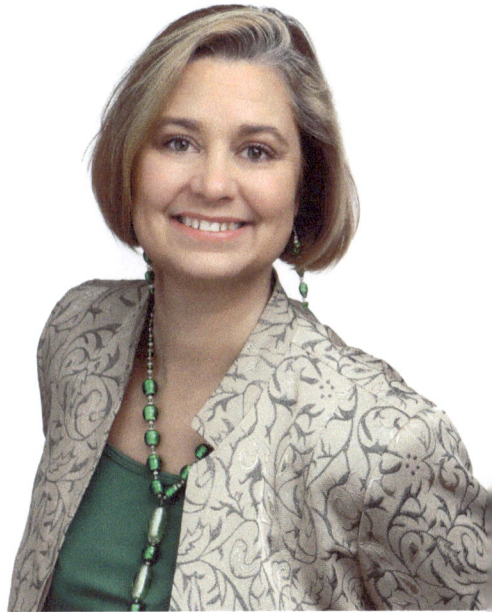

MARIA BERN

Maria is Sara's eldest daughter, is 13 years old. For Maria, it is important to stay healthy and alert.

She has always been keen to learn and contribute to her mother's work. In her leisure time, she plays the piano, acts, rides horses and runs orienteering in the forest.

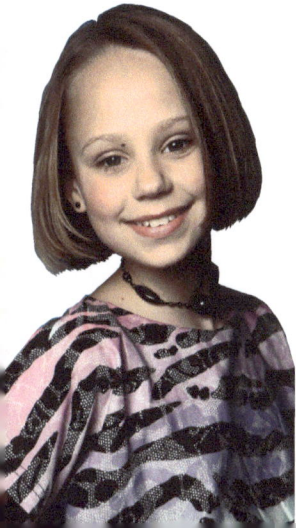

REFERENCES

[i] Victoria Boutenko, *"Green for Life"*, page 75

[ii] Walker WA, Isselbacher KJ. *Uptake and transport of macro-molecules by the intestine. Possible role in clinical disorders.* Gastroenterology: 67:531-50, 1974

[iii] Boutenko, 2010 *"Greens – the Original Source of Omega-3s"*

[iv] *Green for Life* by Victoria Boutenko
http://www.rawfamily.com/recipes
greensmoothiesblog.com/who-is-victoria-boutenko

[v] *60 seconds to slim,* by Michelle Schoffro Cook, PhD, ROHP

[vi] www.care2.com/greenliving/the-top-5-fat-burning-fruits.htlm

[vii] M-P. St-Onge, P.J.H. Jones (2003). *"Greater rise in fat oxidation with medium-chain triglyceride consumption relative to long-chain triglyceride is associated with lower initial body weight and greater loss of subcutaneous adipose tissue".* International Journal of Obesity 27 (12): 1565–1571. doi:10.1038/sj.ijo.0802467. PMID 12975635.

H. Tsuji, M. Kasai, H. Takeuchi, M. Nakamura, M. Okazaki, K. Kondo (2001). *"Dietary Medium-Chain Triacylglycerols Suppress Accumulation of Body Fat in a Double-Blind, Controlled Trial in Healthy Men and Women".* The American Society for Nutritional Sciences 131 (11): 2853–2859. PMID 11694608.

B. Martena, M. Pfeuffer, J. Schrezenmeir (2006). *"Medium-chain triglycerides".* International Dairy Journal 16 (11): 1374–1382. doi:10.1016/j.idairyj.2006.06.015.

Takeuchi, H; Sekine, S; Kojima, K; Aoyama, T (2008). *"The application of medium-chain fatty acids: edible oil with a suppressing effect on body fat accumulation".* Asia Pacific journal of clinical nutrition. 17 Suppl 1: 320–3. PMID 18296368.

St-Onge, MP; Jones, PJ (2002). *"Physiological effects of medium-chain triglycerides: potential agents in the prevention of obesity".* The Journal of nutrition 132 (3): 329–32. PMID 11880549.

[vii] A recent study in the American Journal of Clinical Nutrition indicates that omega-9 fatty acids may play a role in speeding up metabolism and improving mood; *"Substituting dietary monounsaturated fat for saturated fat is associated with increased daily physical activity and resting energy expenditure and with changes in mood."* By Kien CL1, Bunn JY, Tompkins CL, Dumas JA, Crain KI, Ebenstein DB, Koves TR, Muoio DM. Am J Clin Nutr. 2013 Apr;97(4):689-97. doi: 10.3945/ajcn.112.051730. Epub 2013 Feb 27.

[ix] Tomatoes have a lot of vitamin C and the phytochemical lycopene, which stimulates the production of the amino acid known as carnitine. Research shows that carnitine increases the body's fat-burning capacity by one third. Evidence is mounting that carnitine supplements may be beneficial in obesity. The same study showed that in obese rats with insulin resistance, carnitine supplements improved their glucose tolerance and increased the total energy expenditure as well! Pharmacological stimulation of brain carnitine palmitoyl-transferase-1 (CPT-1) was reported to decrease food intake and body weight. And a selective CPT-1 stimulator produced long lasting hypophagia (reduced

food intake) as well as persistent weight loss. Note however, this is in contrast with other studies that found CPT-1 inhibition actually stimulated hypophagia and weight loss. Thus further work needs to be done to clarify this issue.

- Cave MC, Hurt RT, Frazier TH, Matheson PJ, Garrison RN, McClain CJ, McClave SA: *Obesity, inflammation, and the potential application of pharmaconutrition.* Nutr Clin Pract 2008, 23:16-34

- Aja S, Landree LE, Kleman AM, Medghalchi SM, Vadlamudi A, McFadden JM, Aplasca A, Hyun J, Plummer E, Daniels K, Kemm M, Townsend CA, Thupari JN, Kuhajda FP, Moran TH, Ronnett GV: *Pharmacological stimulation of brain carnitine palmitoyl-transferase-1 decreases food intake and body weight.* Am J Physiol Regul Integr Comp Physiol 2008, 294:R352-361.

[xi] *"60 seconds to slim"*, by Michelle Schoffro Cook, PhD, ROHP

[x] The Vitamin C studies:

- U.S. National Library of Medicine: Bromelain. http://www.nlm.nih.gov/medlineplus/druginfo/natural/895.html

- Real Age Medical Encyclopedia: Proteolytic Enzymes http://healthlibrary.epnet.com/GetContent.aspx?token=1edc3d6e-4fec-4b20-baca-795e48830daa&chunkiid=21671

- NutraIngredients.com: Vitamin C Could Lower Body Fat Levels http://www.nutraingredients.com/Research/Vitamin-C-could-lower-body-fat-levels

- Harvard School of Public Health Nutrition Source: Fiber: Start Roughing http://www.hsph.harvard.edu/nutritionsource/what-should-you-eat/fiber-full-story/index.html

- Harvard School of Public Health Nutrition Source: Vegetables and Fruit: The Bottom Line http://www.hsph.harvard.edu/nutritionsource/what-should-you-eat/vegetables-and-fruits/index.html

- American Dietetic Association: Healthy Late Night Snacking http://www.eatright.org/Public/content.aspx?id=6442452691&terms=pineapple

[xi] *IGOB131, a novel seed extract of the West African plant Irvingia gabonensis, significantly reduces body weight and improves metabolic parameters in overweight humans in a randomized double-blind placebo controlled investigation.* Judith L Ngondi, Blanche C Etoundi, Christine B Nyangono, Carl MF Mbofung and Julius E Oben, 2009

[xiii] Help of digestion is also pineapple enzyme bromelain (*4 Strategien*, p.213).

[xiv] *40 Green smoothie recipes for weight loss*, by Jenny Allan

[xiv] *60 seconds to slim*, by Michelle Schoffro Cook, PhD,ROHP and "Grapefruits have a basic alkaline effect after it's digestion" (4 Strategien, p.120)

[xvi] A 2009 study at University of Michigan Cardiovascular Center by researcher E. Mitchell Seymour shows that rats who ate a diet high in blueberries lost abdominal fat -- the kind linked to increased waist size and increased risk for diabetes and heart disease.

[xvii] Federation of American Societies for Experimental Biology (2011, April 10). *Blueberries may inhibit development of fat cells.* ScienceDaily. Retrieved April 10, 2012, from http://www.sciencedaily.com/releases/2011/04/110410130824.htm

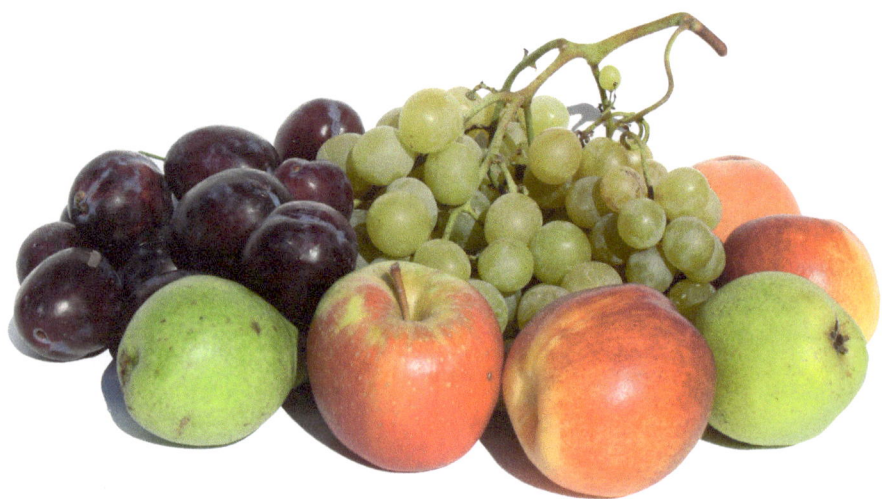